Perpetually Youthful.

"A useful guide for Healthy Aging and Fulfillment"

By

Raquel Ogha

Table of content

Introduction.

In our current world where the quest for youthfulness frequently feels like a relentless race against time, the idea of aging or maturing gracefully feels like an elusive dream. However, concealed inside the folds of time, lies the key to unlocking the true essence of youthfulness - not just in body, but as well as the mind and soul. Welcome to "perpetually Youthful: A Useful Guide for Healthy Aging and Fulfillment," a journey that rises above mere physicality and digs into the profundities of what it means to thrive at each phase of life.

Picture this: a reality where age isn't an obstruction yet an honorable badge, where wrinkles are not indications of shortcoming but rather maps of a life well lived, and where each passing year brings with it insight, vitality, and a renewed feeling of direction. This is the world we welcome you to explore, a reality where the quest for youth isn't about denying nature, but about embracing it earnestly.

As you set out on this journey, you'll find that "perpetually Youthful" isn't simply just another self-improvement guide loaded up with void commitments and handy solutions. All things considered, it's a guide - a commonsense aide created with care and wisdom, intended to engage you to assume command over your well-being, your satisfaction, and your destiny.

Whether you're a young person exploring the wild waters of early adulthood, a seasoned veteran confronting the difficulties of middle age, or a wise elder embracing the brilliant years with effortlessness and respect, there's something here for everybody. Regardless of where you are on life's journey, the mission for fulfillment and vitality is a widespread one.

Anyway, what precisely might you at any point hope to find inside the pages of "Forever Youthful"? Get ready to be propelled, taught, and engaged as we explore a range of topics, including:

1. The Science of Aging: What precisely befalls our bodies as we become older, and how might we saddle the force of science to slow down the aging system and live longer, healthier lives?

2. The Mind-Body connection: Discover the profound ways in which our thoughts, emotions, and beliefs can influence our physical health and well-being, and learn practical techniques for cultivating a positive mindset and reducing

3 Nourishment and Exercise: Explore the most recent exploration on diet and exercise, and figure out what simple lifestyle changes can have a profound impact on our energy levels, temperament, and general vitality.

4. Social Connections: Uncover the importance of social connections and meaningful relationships in advancing longevity and happiness, and learn ways for building and nurturing strong social connections.

5. Purpose and meaning: Dig into the existential questions that lie at the core of the human experience, and find how finding purpose and meaning in life can enhance our sense of fulfillment and well-being.

6. Embracing Change: Learn to embrace the certainty of progress and explore life's advances with elegance and versatility, whether it's starting a new career, facing retirement, or coping with loss and grief.

7. The power of gratitude: Develop an attitude of gratitude and appreciation for the blessings in your day-to-day living, and find how practicing appreciation can change your perspective and improve your general sense of well-being.

All through your journey with "perpetually Youthful," you'll experience genuine accounts of people who have defined the odds, defeated difficulty, and embraced the magnificence of aging with boldness and effortlessness. From centenarians who keep on flourishing great into their brilliant years to youthful grown-ups who are reclassifying growing old, their accounts act as a strong wake-up call that age is only a number - and that the genuine mystery to timeless youth exists in all of us.

All in all, would you say you are prepared to leave on this extraordinary journey? Could it be said that you are prepared to embrace the force of aging with elegance, vitality, and purpose? Provided that this is true, then turn the page and let the experience start. Welcome to "perpetually Youthful: A Viable Guide for healthy Aging and

Fulfillment" - where age is only a number, and the best is on way..

Chapter One

Unraveling the Secrets of Aging.

In the core of a clamoring city, in the midst of the buzzing about day-to-day existence, there carried on with a lady named Clara. At 85 years old, Clara was an awe-inspiring phenomenon - her silver hair sparkling in the daylight, her eyes gleaming with youthfulness and her chuckling ringing out like music in the air. To the people who knew her, Clara was the embodiment of vitality and beauty, a living testament of the force of maturing with fulfillment and enthusiasm.

Yet, Clara wasn't generally the lively, fiery soul that she is today. In the same way as other of us, she once dreaded the progression of time, fearing the unavoidable walk of kinks and silver hairs that would check the years gone by. However, as she ventured through life's exciting bends in the road, Clara came to understand that maturing was not something to be feared, but something to be embraced - a journey of self-discovery and change that held the way to opening life's most prominent secrets.

As Clara sat in her comfortable loft, sipping tea and looking out at the world underneath, she wanted to wonder about the miracle, all things considered. How is it, she pondered, that certain individuals appear to mature with effortlessness and vitality, while others surrender to the ravages of time? What mysteries lie concealed inside the depths of our cells, ready to be found?

To unravel the secrets of aging, Clara left on a quest for knowledge, drenching herself in the most recent exploration and discoveries. What she found was both captivating and enlightening, challenging the preconceived notion of what the world holds about becoming old.

Aging isn't just about wrinkles and silver hairs - a complex biological process that influences every part of our body, from the tips of our toes to the depths of our soul. At its core, aging is driven by a myriad of factors, including hereditary qualities, lifestyle choices, and environmental factors, all of which connect in complicated ways to shape our journey through life.

One of the key players in the aging process is something many refer to as telomeres - tiny caps at the end of our chromosomes that shield our DNA from damage. As we age, our telomeres gradually shortens, leading to cellular aging and an increased risk of age-related illnesses. Yet, here's the intriguing part: research has shown that specific way of life factors like Exercise ,stress management , and healthy diet choices can actually slow down the rate of telomere shortening, allowing us to age more gracefully and maintain our youthful vitality for longer.

Yet, aging isn't just about science - it's also about mindset. As Clara found on her journey, our convictions and perspectives towards aging can significantly affect how we experience the passage of time. Assuming we view aging as a natural and inescapable part of life, instead of something to be feared or resisted, we can move toward each passing year with a sense of curiosity and wonder, embracing the wisdom and experience that accompanies age.

Take, for instance, the tale of Henry, a resigned teacher who went through his brilliant years venturing to the far corners of the planet and seeking after his enthusiasm for photography. Despite his advancing age, Henry moved toward each new experience with the excitement and energy of a young fellow, refusing to allow his age define him or cut off his true capacity. What's more, in doing so, he found that age isn't a hindrance to making every second count - it's a gift, a valuable chance to explore, grow, and connect with the world around us..

As Clara dug further into the mysteries of aging, she understood that there is no size-fits-all solution to growing old smoothly. Instead , it's a journey of self-discovery and exploration, a mission to reveal the mysteries of longevity and vitality that exist in all of us. Whether we're eighty-five or twenty-Five we all have the power to shape our fates and embrace the beauty of aging with grace, beauty, and vitality

Thus, as you set out on your journey through the sands of life, recall this: aging isn't a curse, but a gift - an opportunity to enjoy the wealth of life and find the genuine meaning of fulfillment. Embrace each passing year with open arms, and let the wonder of it guide you on the path to staying youthful. After all, as Clara would agree, age is only a number - and the best is on the way.

Chapter Two.

Nourishing Your Body: The Groundwork of Health and Vitality.

In the buzzing of our everyday life, it's easy to overlook one of the most fundamental parts of taking care of oneself: nourishing our bodies is simple. However, the food we eat assumes a basic part in energizing our actual energy as well as in supporting our mental clarity, emotional wellness and overall vitality. In this exploration of nourishment, we'll dig into the significance of making mindful food choices, cultivating a healthy relationship with food, and embracing the transformative power of nourishing our bodies from the back to the front.

Understanding Nutrition:

At its center, nutrition is the study of how food nourishes our bodies, giving us the essential nutrient required for growth, repair, and optimal functioning.These nutrients include carbohydrates, proteins, fats, nutrients, minerals, and water, each assuming a remarkable part in supporting our health and well-being.

Carbohydrates act as our body's primary source of energy, energizing everything from our morning rush to our early evening time meetings to generate new ideas. Proteins are the structural blocks of life, fundamental for muscle development, tissue fix, and immune function. Fats provides us with a concentrated source of energy, as well as assuming a fundamental part in chemical creation and cell membrane integrity

Nutrients and minerals go about as co -factors in endless biochemical responses all through the body, supporting everything from bone health to immune function to energy metabolism. What's more, water - the remedy of life - is fundamental for keeping up with hydration, controlling internal heat levels, and flushing out toxins.

- ## The Force of Careful Eating

In a universe of fast food and fad diets, the idea of careful eating offers a refreshing alternate - a re-visitation of simplicity, balance, and presence in our relationship with food. Careful eating is about something beyond what we eat - it's about how we eat ,when we eat, and why we eat.

By slowing down and enjoying each nibble, we can take advantage of the sensory experience of eating - the texture, flavors, and smells that make food such a rich and remunerating part of life. By focusing on our body's appetite and fullness cues, we can figure out how to eat in arrangement with our regular craving and satiety signals, rather than external cues   or emotional triggers.

Careful eating likewise welcomes us to develop a more profound familiarity with the connection between our food decisions and our general well-being   and   vitality.   Heather   than approaching food as a means to an end - whether that   is   weight   reduction,   performance optimization, or emotional comfort - we can see it   as   a   source   of   nourishment   and   delight, respecting our body's unique needs and preferences with each and every meal.

Embracing whole Foods

In a world dominated by processed, convenience food, the simple act of embracing natural food sources can be an extreme demonstration of taking care of oneself. Whole food sources - like organic products, vegetables, entire grains, vegetables, nuts, seeds, and lean proteins - are loaded with the supplements our bodies need to flourish, without the additional sugars, additives, and counterfeit added substances seen in many processed food sources.

By focusing on whole food in our eating routine, we can fuel our bodies with the nutrients, minerals, cell reinforcements, and phytonutrients expected to help ideal well-being and vitality. From the lively shades of new products of the soil to the generous decency of whole grains and vegetables, natural food varieties offer a symphony of flavors and textures that can support our bodies as well as our spirits.

- **Creating balance and variety**

While whole food varieties structure the underpinning of a healthy diet, embracing balance and variety in our food choices is likewise significant. Rather than fixing a specific nutrient or slandering entire food groups, we can approach a flexible and comprehensive way to deal with eating that honors the diverse needs and preferences of our bodies.

This could mean enjoying a colorful array of fruits and vegetables at each meal, incorporating a variety of protein sources like beans, lentils, tofu, fish, and poultry, and exploring different avenues regarding various grains, nuts, seeds, and flavors to add depth and flavor to our meals.

It likewise implies being mindful of portion sizes and checking out our body's craving and fullness cues to direct our eating patterns. By striking a balance between nourishment and pleasure, we can make a sustainable and fulfilling way to deal with eating that upholds our well-being and vitality for the long haul.

- **The Transformative Force of Nourishment**

Ultimately, nourishing our bodies is about something other than powering our physical energy - it's tied in with nurturing our psyche, body, and soul in an all-encompassing and coordinated manner. At the point when we approach food with respect and regard, we tap into a deep well of wisdom and vitality that can change our relationship with ourselves and our general surroundings.

From the basic demonstration of relishing a piece of ripe fruit to the delight of sharing a meal with friends and family, with each bite we make a move to nourish ourselves on a significant level - to renew our energy, recharge our spirits, and replenish our connection with the natural world.

Thus, as you explore the journey of feeding your body, recollect this: food isn't simply fuel - it's medication, it's pleasure, it's fellowship. Embrace the force of careful eating, whole food sources, balance, and variety, and let the transformative force of nourishment guide you on the way to brilliant well-being and vitality.

All things considered, when we feed our bodies, we support our spirits - and the conceivable outcomes are huge

Nutrition for longevity: fuelling Your Body for an Energetic Life

Introduction:

As we continue looking for a long and satisfying life, nutrition remains one of the most useful assets available to us. The food we eat has the capacity not only to nourish our bodies but also to help our well-being, vitality, and life span. In this exploration of nourishment for longevity we'll dig into the study of aging, the job of nutrition in advancing life span, and down-to-earth systems for energizing your body for a dynamic and satisfying life.

- *Grasping the Study of Aging*

Aging is a mind-boggling and diverse interaction that influences each part of our being, from the cellular level to our overall health and well-being. While aging is impacted by various elements, including hereditary qualities, way of life, and environmental influences, one of the vital drivers of aging is something many refer to as oxidative stress.

Oxidative stress happens when there is an imbalance between free radicals - unstable molecules that can harm cells and DNA - and cancer prevention agents, which help to kill these harmful molecules. After some time, these combined harmful molecules can add to the aging system and increase the rate of age-related illnesses like coronary illness, disease, and neurodegenerative problems.

Luckily, the food varieties we eat contain an abundance of cell reinforcements, nutrients, minerals, and phytonutrients that can assist with combatting oxidative pressure and backing sound maturing. By integrating supplement-rich food varieties into our eating routine, we can sustain our bodies from the back to front, advancing life span and vitality into our brilliant years.

- ***The Job of Nutrition in Advancing Longevity***

With regards to advancing life span, the familiar saying "you are what you eat" sounds accurate. The food sources we devour consistently assume a basic part in molding our well-being and health, impacting everything from our energy levels to our mental capability to our defenselessness to ongoing illnesses.

Research has shown that specific dietary patterns -, for example, the Mediterranean diet, which is rich in fruit, vegetables, entire grains, fish, nuts, and olive oil - are related to a lower rate of chronic disease and a long life span. These dietary patterns are rich in fundamental nutrients and antioxidants as well as low in processed food varieties, refined sugars, and unhealthy fats that can add to aggravation and oxidative pressure.

As well as advancing life span, a nutrient-rich eating routine can likewise improve quality of life as we age, supporting solid aging by protecting mental capability, keeping up with bulk and strength, and diminishing the risk of age-related incapacities.

- ***Practical strategies for fuelling your body for Longevity.***

All in all, how might you fuel your body for a long and dynamic life? Here are a few practical strategies to assist you with getting everything rolling:

1. Eat colorful fruit and vegetables.

Fill your plate with different beautiful colors of fruits and vegetables, which are loaded with nutrients, minerals, antioxidants, and phytonutrients that help in overall health and well-being.

2. Pick whole, Natural Food varieties.

Choose whole grains, lean proteins, healthy fats, and vegetables, which give a rich source of essential nutrients without the preservatives, additives, and counterfeit added substances tracked down in many handled food sources.

3. Focus on Omega-3 Unsaturated fats.
Incorporate wellsprings of omega-3 unsaturated fats, like fatty fish (salmon, mackerel, sardines), flaxseeds, chia seeds, and walnuts, which have been displayed to help heart well-being, mind capability, and overall health and well-being.

4. Limit Added Sugars and processed foods

Limit your intake of added sugars, refined carbohydrates, and processed food, which can add to irritation, oxidative stress, and an increased rate of chronic disease.

5. Stay hydrated: Drink a lot of water over the day to remain hydrated and support optimal body functions, like assimilation, digestion, and detoxification.

6. Stay active: in addition to a healthy diet, one must stay active by exercising regularly to promote longevity and vitality. Aim for at least 150 minutes of moderate-intensive exercise per week, like brisk walking, swimming, cycling, or dancing.

- **Conclusion**

In the journey of life, nutrition serves as a compass, directing us toward a way of health, well-being, and vitality. By nourishing our bodies with nutrient-rich foods, we can support healthy aging, enhance quality of life, and open the maximum capacity of our physical, mental, and emotional well-being.

Thus, as you leave to embark on your journey toward longevity, remember this: the decisions and choices you make today have the ability to shape your health and vitality for years to come. Embrace the transformative power of nutrition, fuel your body with intention and purpose, and appreciate the journey of living your longest, healthiest, and most vibrant life possible.

-
- **Exercise for vitality: Harnessing the power of movement for optimal well-being.**

Introduction.

In the journey for vitality and well-being, scarcely anything is as potent as the transformative power of exercise. Movement isn't just about sculpting a toned physique or shedding undesirable pounds - it's tied in with supporting our bodies, empowering our spirits, and opening the maximum capacity of our physical, mental, and emotional well-being. In this exploration of exercise for vitality, we'll dive into the science of movement, the advantages of ordinary physical activities, and practical techniques for integrating exercise into your day-to-day routine to flourish and thrive

- ***Grasping the science of movement:***

At its core, exercise is a type of physical activity that engages our muscles, joints, and cardiovascular system, promoting strength, adaptability, perseverance, and generally physical fitness. However, the advantages of benefits of exercise go a long way past the actual domain - research has demonstrated the way that regular physical activity can likewise significantly affect our psychological and emotional well-being, upgrading our state of mind, lessening stress, and working on mental capability.

At the point when we work out, our bodies discharge hormones and neurotransmitters - including endorphins, serotonin, and dopamine - that promote feelings of pleasure, happiness, and relaxation. These natural mood boosters can assist with mitigating side symptoms of uneasiness and sadness, improve confidence and self-perception, and develop a more noteworthy feeling of overall well-being.

- ***The Advantages and benefits of regular physical exercise.***

The benefits of regular physical exercise are far-reaching, influencing virtually every part of health and well-being. From lessening the risk of chronic diseases to improving sleep quality to improving mental capability, exercise offers an abundance of advantages that can assist us with flourishing at each phase of life.

Physical health: Regular exercise has been shown to reduce the risk of chronic diseases like heart disease, type 2 diabetes, and certain types of cancer. It can likewise assist with bringing down blood pressure, further develop cholesterol levels, and support healthy weight management.

Emotional and Mental health: Exercise effectively affects emotional well-being, lessening side effects of uneasiness and discouragement, anxiety further developing the mindset, and improving by and large mental well-being. It can likewise assist with mitigating stress, boost confidence, and advance better sleep quality.

Cognitive Function: Research has shown that regular physical activity can have profound effects on cognitive function, improving memory, attention, and executive function. Exercise may also help to reduce the risk of age-related cognitive decline and neurodegenerative diseases such as Alzheimer's disease.

Practical Strategies for Incorporating Exercise into Your Life:

All in all, how can you harness the power of exercise to enhance your vitality and well-being? Here are a few practical strategies to assist you with getting everything rolling:

1. Find Exercises You Appreciate: Exercise doesn't need to be a task - it very well may be a wellspring of happiness, joy, and satisfaction. Explore different avenues regarding various kinds of exercise until you find something you truly appreciate, whether it's climbing, dancing, swimming, cycling, or practicing martial arts.

2. Set realistic goals: Begin little, then step by step move toward difficult exercises as your fitness level improves. Set reasonable, attainable objectives that line up with your inclinations, and capacities, and commend your progress along the way.

3. Make It Social: Exercise is many times more enjoyable when finished with others, so why not enroll the help of companions, relatives, or exercise pals to go along with you on your fitness journey Whether it's joining a games group, going to a gathering fitness class, or taking a stroll with a companion, practicing with others can assist with keeping you motivated, responsible, and accountable.

4. Focus on Consistency: Consistency is key with regards to benefiting the rewards of exercise, so expect to make physical activity a regular part of your day to day daily practice. Track down valuable chances to integrate development into your everyday life, whether it's using the stairwell rather than the lift, strolling or trekking to work, or planning standard exercise meetings into your schedule.

5. Stand by listening to Your Body: Focus on your body's signs and change your workout routine likewise. In a situation when you're feeling drained or sore, allow yourself to rest and recuperate. Also, assuming that you're feeling energized and inspired, seize the opportunity to challenge yourself and stretch your boundaries.

Conclusion

Exercise isn't just about building an ideal physique or accomplishing particular fitness goals - it's tied in with embracing the delight of movement, nurturing our bodies, and opening the maximum capacity of our physical, mental, and emotional well-being. By incorporating regular physical activity into our lives, we can enhance our vitality, boost our temperament, and flourish at each phase of life. So lace up your sneakers, find exercises that give you pleasure, and embark on a journey of movement, vitality, and well-being that will enrich your life for years to come.

Sleep and Restorative Pratices: unlocking the Mending power of Rest.

Introduction:

In a world that never appears to slow down, the worth of rest and restorative practices frequently gets ignored. However, underneath our hectic lives lies a significant truth: rest isn't simply a luxury, but a fundamental human need - a period for our bodies and psyches to rest, fix, and revive. In this exploration of rest and restorative practices, we'll dive into the study of rest, the significance of rest for overall health and vitality, and practical techniques for developing a deep sense of relaxation and renewal in our daily lives.

- **Grasping the science of Rest.**

Rest is a mind-boggling and dynamic cycle that assumes a crucial part in essentially every part of our well-being and vitality. During rest, our bodies go through different physiological and neurological changes that support physical repair, cognitive function, emotional processing, and immune function.

One of the key stages of sleep is Rapid eye movement (REM) rest, during which our brains become exceptionally active, and we experience distinctive dreams. REM sleep is thought to assume a pivotal part in memory consolidation, emotional regulation, and learning.

One more significant phase of sleep is non-REM sleep, which is characterized by slower brain waves and deeper relaxation. Non-REM sleep is essential for physical relaxation, hormone regulation, and overall rejuvenation of the body.

- **The Significance of Restorative Practices**

In addition to sleep, restorative practices envelop many exercises and techniques that promote relaxation, stress reduction, and inner peace. These practices can incorporate mindfulness meditation, deep breathing exercises, moderate muscle relaxation, and guided imagery.

The advantages of Restorative practices are manifold, stretching out past the physical realm to envelop mental, emotional, and spiritual well-being. By engaging in regular restorative practices, we can reduce stress, improve sleep quality, enhance our state of mind, and develop a more prominent feeling of balance and harmony in our lives.

- **Practical strategies for cultivating rest.**

Anyway, how might you integrate helpful practices into your everyday daily schedule to advance relaxation and renewal? Here are a few practical steps to assist you with getting everything rolling:

1. Create a relaxing bedtime routine

Sleep Schedule: Lay out a relieving sleep time routine to indicate to your body that now is the ideal time to slow down and plan for rest. This could incorporate exercises like having a warm or cold bath, reading a book, practicing gentle stretching exercises, or listening to calming music.

2. Limit exposure to Screens: Limit exposure to electronic gadgets -, for example, cell phones, tablets, PCs, and TVs - in the hour leading to bedtime, as the blue light transmitted by these gadgets can disrupt the production of melatonin, a hormone that controls sleep-wake cycles.

3. Practice mindfulness Meditation:

Set aside time every day to practice mindfulness meditation, a simple yet strong practice that includes concentrating on the present moment without judgment. Mindfulness meditation has been shown to reduce pressure or stress, further develop sleep quality, and upgrade general well-being.

4. Attempt Progressive Muscle Relaxation:

Progressive Muscle Relaxation is a relaxation method that includes straining and afterward releasing each muscle group in the body, one at a time. This can help with lessening muscle tension, enhance relaxation, and set up the body for rest.

5. Practice deep Breathing Exercises: Deep breathing exercises, for example, diaphragmatic breathing or the 4-7-8 method, can assist with activating the body's relaxation response, lower feelings of anxiety, and enhance sensations of quiet and peacefulness.

6. Create a Tranquil Sleep Environment: Make your room a haven for sleep by establishing a serene and agreeable environment. This could include investing in a comfortable mattress and pillows, shutting out external noise with earplugs or repetitive sound, and guaranteeing that the room is cool, dim, and free from distractions.

- **Conclusion.**

In a world that appears to move constantly, the worth of sleep and restorative practices couldn't possibly be more overstated. By focusing on rest and integrating regular restorative practices into our day-to-day routines, we can nurture our bodies, soothe our minds, and develop a deeper sense of well-being and vitality. So take the time to rest, rejuvenate, and reconnect with the healing power of adequate rest. Your body, mind, and soul will be thankful for it.

Chapter Three

Developing a Sharp Psyche for Timeless Youth.

Introduction:
In the pursuit of being forever youthful, one of the most neglected at this point is the development of a sharp psyche. While physical health and well-being frequently become the dominant focal point, keeping up with mental nimbleness and smartness is similarly critical for keeping up with being healthy. In this chapter, we will dive into the importance of developing a sharp brain with regards to being youthful, exploring different methodologies, activities, and exercises that advance mental well-being and life span.

- ## **Understanding the significance of mental sharpness.**

A sharp psyche isn't just about knowledge or academic achievement - it's about mental spryness, mental adaptability, and emotional resilience. As we age, our minds go through changes that can influence memory, consideration, and critical thinking skills. Nonetheless, by effectively engaging in activities that stimulate our brains, we can keep up with mental capability and avoid age-related decline.

Research has shown that people who routinely challenge their minds through exercises like reading, puzzles, and deep-rooted learning have a lower risk of developing mental degradation and dementia. By keeping our psyches active and engaged, we can maintain cognitive function and enhance our overall quality of life as we age.

- ### *Mental Wellness Exercise*

Mental wellness practices are like exercises for our brains, assisting with keeping them sharp, agile, and strong. These activities challenge various parts of mental capability, including memory, attention, and critical thinking abilities. How about we explore some compelling mental wellness works out:

1. Crossword Riddles and Sudoku: These exemplary riddles are astounding for stimulating critical thinking abilities and memory. By regularly engaging in crossword riddles and Sudoku, we can keep our psyches sharp and agile while having a great time.

2. Brain teasers and Riddles: Entertaining riddles and conundrums challenge our critical thinking abilities and decisive reasoning skills. These riddles expect us to think creatively and fresh, which assists with keeping our psyches sharp and flexible.

3. Memory Games: Memory games, like matching games or concentration, are perfect for practicing our memory and ability to focus. These games can assist with working on our capacity to hold and review data, which is fundamental for keeping up with mental capability as we age.

4. Mindfulness Meditation: mindfulness meditation includes concentrating on the present moment without judgment. This training has been displayed to reduce stress, further develop concentration, and improve general well-being. By infusing mindfulness meditation into our everyday daily routine, we can prepare our brains to be more present and attentive.

- ***Stimulating brain activities***

I'm addition to mental wellness works out, taking part in stimulating brain activities is fundamental for keeping our brains sharp and vibrant. These exercises challenge our brains in previously unheard-of ways, advancing brain adaptability and mental versatility. We should explore some stimulating brain exercises:

1. **Learning Another/New Skill:** Whether it's playing an instrument, learning another dialect, or mastering another hobby, learning a new skill is a brilliant method for stimulating our minds and brains. These exercises challenge us to step beyond our usual ranges of familiarity and participate in continuous learning, which is fundamental for keeping up with mental capability.

2. **Puzzle Games and Strategy Games:** Puzzle games and strategy games, like chess or Scrabble, are perfect for stimulating our minds

and enhancing cognitive function. These games expect us to plan, prepare, and think logically, which can assist with working on mental capability and critical thinking abilities.

3. Artistic Expression: Participating in creative exercises, like composition, drawing, or chiseling, can stimulate creativity and promote emotional well-being. These exercises urge us to articulate our thoughts innovatively and can assist with working on our temperament and reducing stress.

5. Physical Exercise: Physical Exercise isn't just advantageous for our bodies but also helps with our brain. Regular exercise has been displayed to work on mental capability, enhance memory, and reduce the risk of mental degradation. Exercises like strolling and swimming can assist with keeping our psyches sharp and lithe.

- *Importance of life-long learning*.

Life-long learning is the foundation of remaining everlastingly youthful and young, furnishing us with potential open doors for self-awareness, intellectual stimulation, and emotional fulfillment. The quest for information keeps our psyches dynamic and connected, cultivating interest, innovativeness, and a feeling of miracle. We should explore the significance of life-lifelong learning:

1. Intellectual stimulation: Lifelong learning challenges us to explore new ideas, viewpoints, and experiences, stimulating our psyches and growing our points of view. Whether it's reading a book, attending lectures, or taking a class, long-lasting learning keeps our minds dynamic and engaged, promoting mental well-being and vitality.

2. Self-awareness: Long-lasting learning gives us open doors for self-awareness and advancement. By constantly seeking out new knowledge and skills, we can develop a growth mindset and embrace the difficulties and challenges that come our direction.

3. Adaptability: In the present fast-paced world, the capacity to adjust to change is more important than at any time in recent memory. Long-lasting learning assists us with remaining agile and versatile, equipping us with the skills and knowledge expected to explore life's exciting bend with certainty and resilience.

4.   Emotional   Fulfillment: Long-lasting learning improves our lives and presents us with a feeling of satisfaction and fulfillment. Whether it's learning another language, mastering an instrument, or exploring a new hobby, life-long learning permits us to seek after our passion and interests, giving us pleasure and bliss.

Developing a sharp brain is essential for staying everlastingly youthful, both intellectually and inwardly. By taking part in mental wellness works, stimulating brain activities, and embracing the life-long quest for learning, we can keep our brains and minds sharp, agile, and vibrant all through our lives. So let us focus on supporting our psyches, expanding our horizons, and embracing the journey of aging.

- **Developing a Sharp Psyche by having sufficient rest**

In addition to specific mental activities and stimulating exercises, developing a sharp psyche likewise includes embracing day-to-day activities that help mental well-being and vitality. These habits might appear to be little, however, their combined effect can be huge in keeping up with smartness and advancing long-lasting learning.

1. Get Satisfactory Rest: Quality rest is fundamental for mental capability and generally speaking mental well-being. During rest, the brain consolidates memories, processes information, and flushes out toxins. Aim for 7-9 hours of restful sleep every night to support optimal brain function.

2. Stay physical activity: Regular physical activity helps the body as well as the mind. Exercise increases blood flow to the brain, stimulates the release of growth factors, and improves neuroplasticity - the mind's capacity to adapt and reorganize. Incorporate exercises you enjoy, like strolling, dancing, or swimming, into your day-to-day routine to keep both your body and psyche in top shape.

3. Eat a Brain-Healthy Diet: Nourishment assumes a basic part in mental well-being, so fuel your body with food sources that help mental capability. Center around a reasonable eating routine rich in fruits, vegetables, whole grains, lean proteins, and healthy fats. Omega-3 unsaturated fats, found in fatty fish, nuts, and seeds, are especially gainful for mental well-being.

4. Remain Socially Connected: Social communication is indispensable for mental health and emotional well-being. Participate in important discussions, and maintain close relationships with loved ones. Socializing stimulates the brain, supports the state of mind, and decreases the risk of mental deterioration.

5. Challenge Your Mind: Keep your brain sharp by persistently testing yourself with new challenges and activities. Try learning another dialect, playing an instrument, or handling a complex puzzle. Novel encounters stimulate the mind and promote the growth of new neural connections.

6. Practice Mindfulness: Mindfulness practices, like meditation and deep breathing exercises, can help reduce stress, further develop concentration, and improve mental capability. Set aside opportunity every day to calm your brain, focus on your breath, and develop a feeling of inward harmony and clarity.

7. Stay Curious: Cultivate an inquisitive mindset by staying open to new ideas, experiences, and perspectives. Ask questions, explore new interests, and search out potential open doors for learning and development. An inquisitive mind is a flexible mind, equipped for adapting to new challenges and embracing long-lasting learning.

- ***Overpowering Hindrances to Mental Sharpness:***

While developing a sharp brain is significant, it's not always easy, and there might be obstructions that ruin our endeavors. Recognizing and addressing these obstructions is critical to keeping up with mental health and vitality.

1. Stress: chronic stress can negatively affect mental capability, and weaken memory, attention, and critical thinking abilities. Practice stress management strategies like deep breathing, mindfulness meditation, and physical exercise to reduce feelings of anxiety and support brain health.

2. Sedentary lifestyle: An inactive way of life can adversely influence mental capability and increase the risk of mental deterioration. Try to integrate regular physical activity into your day-to-day daily schedule, regardless of whether it's simply a short walk or a gentle stretching session.

3. Poor Nutrition: A diet high in processed foods, sugar, and undesirable fats can impede mental capability and add to mental deterioration. Focus on eating a balanced diet rich in fruits, vegetables, whole grains, lean proteins, and healthy fats to support brain health.

4 Absence of sleep: Sleep deprivation can significantly affect mental capability, impairing memory, concentration, and critical thinking skills. Prioritize sleep and lay out a healthy rest timetable to guarantee you get the rest your brain needs to ideally work.

5. Social Isolation: Social confinement can adversely affect mental well-being and vitality. Try to remain connected with others, whether through in-person interactions, calls, or video talks. Join clubs, volunteer gatherings, or social associations to cultivate meaningful connections and battle loneliness.

Conclusion.

In the journey for eternal youth, developing a sharp psyche is fundamental for keeping up with mental well-being, vitality, and overall well-being. By engaging in mental wellness works, stimulating brain activities, taking on everyday habits that help mental well-being, and overcoming barriers to mental sharpness, we can keep our psyches agile, strong, and forever youthful. So let us focus on nurturing our psyches, extending our viewpoints, and embracing the journey of long-lasting learning - for in the pursuit of knowledge lies the way to everlasting youth.

Chapter Four

Nurturing Your Spirit.

Introduction

In the pursuit of staying youthful, it's essential not only to focus on your physical well-being alone but also focus on nurturing your spirit - the essence of what our identity is. Developing inward vitality and emotional well-being is key to living a satisfying and energetic life at any stage in life. In this chapter, we will explore the importance of nourishing your spirit with regard to healthy aging and life-long satisfaction, looking at different practices, standards, and perspectives that improve inward growth, versatility, and joy.

- *Understanding the word "Spirit"*

The spirit is often depicted as the substance of our being - the piece of us that rises above the physical body and connects us with something greater than ourselves. While it can be challenging to define or quantify, nurturing our spirit involves cultivating attitudes like gratitude, empathy, resilience, and inner peace. By keeping an eye on our emotional well-being, we can experience greater meaning, purpose, and satisfaction in our lives.

• Practices for Nurturing Our Spirit

1. Gratitude Practice: cultivating an attitude of gratitude can profoundly affect our spiritual well-being. By taking time every day to reflect on the things we are thankful for, we can move our perspective from lack to abundance, cultivating a feeling of satisfaction, happiness, and gratitude for life's blessings.

2. Self-compassion: Practicing self-compassion includes treating ourselves with kindness, understanding, and acceptance, particularly during times of challenges. By offering ourselves the same sympathy and compassion we would give to a friend, we can develop more prominent strength, self-acknowledgment, and emotional well-being.

3. Connecting with Nature: Spending time in nature can be a source of nourishment for our spirit and soul, helping us with a feeling of being associated with something greater than ourselves and helping us to remember the excellence and wonder of the natural world. Whether it's going for a hike, taking a walk in the park, or just sitting outside and absorbing the sights and hints of nature, these can help restore a feeling of peace and harmony.

- ● *Standards for Nurturing Your Spirit*

1. Authenticity: Nurturing the spirit requires genuineness - the courage to be true to ourselves, embrace our strengths and weaknesses, and live in alignment with our values and aspirations. At the point we like genuinely, we develop a deeper sense of self-awareness, integrity, and inner peace.

2. Compassion: compassion is the heart of spiritual growth, cultivating compassion, generosity, and connections with others. By developing a compassionate attitude towards ourselves as well as other people, we create an expanding influence of healing, understanding, and love that nourishes the soul and fosters greater harmony and unity in the world.

3. Resilience: Resilience is the ability to bounce back from difficulty, overcome challenges, and grow stronger in the process. Nurturing the spirit involves developing resilience - the capacity to confront life's highs and lows with boldness, effortlessness, and resilience, realizing that we have the inward resources and strength to navigate whatever comes our direction.

4. Gratitude: Gratitude is a fundamental spiritual practice that develops a feeling of abundance, gratitude, and satisfaction throughout everyday life. By cultivating an attitude of gratitude, we shift our focus from what is lacking and thankful for what is present, encouraging a deep feeling of satisfaction, fulfillment, and well-being.

- *The role of spirituality in healthy aging.*

Spirituality plays a huge role in healthy maturing and aging, providing a source of strength, meaning, and resilience as we navigate the challenges and transitions of later life. Research has shown that people who have a strong sense of spirituality or connection with something greater than themselves tend to experience greater psychological well-being, lower levels of stress, and better overall health outcomes.

Conclusion

In the pursuit of being forever youthful, nourishing your spirit is essential for cultivating inward vitality, versatility, and satisfaction. By practicing mindfulness, self-compassion, and creativity, and embracing standards like geniuses, empathy, and resilience, we can nourish our spirits and develop a more profound feeling of meaning, purpose, and well-being in our lives. So let us commit to tending to our spiritual well-being, connecting with our innermost selves, and embracing the journey of self-discovery and growth - for in the nourishing of our spirits lies the path to living a vibrant and fulfilling life at any stage in life.

- ***Connections and Community Engagement***

Maintaining strong social connections with your community is an essential factor for healthy aging and fulfillment. Social interactions provide emotional support, reduce feelings of loneliness and isolation, and promote overall well-being.

Here are some ways to nurture social connections and engage with your community.

1. Stay active in social circles

Try to stay connected with companions, family, and friends. Go to parties, organize trips, and set up regular meetups to keep up with meaningful relationships. Whether it's hosting a dinner gathering, taking a stroll with a friend, or joining a book club, find opportunities to connect with others and support your social network.

2. Join Clubs or Gatherings

Joining clubs or gatherings with similar interests can give amazing open doors to social interactions and community engagement. Whether it's a hobby club, sports group, or community organization, taking part in such exercises allows you to meet new individuals, share experiences, and build connections based on common interests.

3. Volunteer and give back.

Taking part in humanitarian work or community service activity isn't just a method for impacting your community but also a means of connecting with others and finding purpose and fulfillment. Volunteer at local communities, schools, or non-profit groups that align with your interests and values. Whether it's tutoring students, or participating in environmental clean-up efforts, find ways of giving back to your community and making a positive impact.

4. Participate in Educational and Recreational Activities

Take part in educational and recreational activities that encourage social connections and self-growth. Take classes or studios on points that interest you, like workmanship, cooking, music, or wellness. Join sporting games associations or wellness gatherings to meet new individuals and remain dynamic while having some good times. These exercises furnish chances to connect and relate with other people who share your passion and interests, encouraging friendship.

5. Have Get-togethers

Step up and have get-togethers and occasions at your home or in your community. Whether it's a potluck dinner, game night, or lawn grill, facilitating get-togethers allows you to unite individuals and make memorable experiences. Welcome friends, family, neighbors, and colleagues to share food, giggling, and discussion, strengthening bonds and fostering a sense of belonging.

6. Support and Empower Others

Be a source of help and support for others in your group of friends and community. Offer a listening ear, encouraging words, or commonsense help to those in need. Volunteer to help friends or neighbors with errands, for example, shopping for food, home fixes, or transportation. By offering love and sympathy towards others, you reinforce your social connections as well as add to a culture of caring and reciprocity within your community.

7. Stay informed and engaged in community issues.

Remain informed about local and worldwide issues that influence your community and the world at large. Go to local gatherings, municipal centers, and gatherings to keep up to date with recent developments and take part in it, participate in conversations about relevant. By effectively engaging in community issues, you add to positive change and strengthen the fabric of your community while connecting with other people who share your values and concerns.

8. Celebrate Milestones and Accomplishments

Find opportunities to celebrate achievements, accomplishments, and exceptional feats with friends, family, and community members. Whether it's a birthday, anniversary, graduation, or retirement, mark these moments with joy and gratitude, surrounded by friends and family. Have festivities, gatherings, or social occasions to honor these significant achievements and make lasting memories together. Commending life's achievements cultivates a feeling of connection, appreciation, and kinship among loved ones, reinforcing bonds and deepening relationships.

By effectively taking part in social connections and community engagement, you enrich your life with meaningful connections, shared experiences, and a feeling of belonging. Whether it's through get-togethers, voluntary work, intergenerational projects, or community engagement, prioritize activities that nurture connection and encourage a feeling of belonging. By doing so, you do not just support your well-being and fulfillment, but also add to the general benefit of the society, creating a

more vibrant and connected community for individuals, of all ages, to thrive in.

Chapter Five

"Embracing Change"

Let's explore this with storytelling, as we go on a ride on how to embrace change, it promises to be captivating, relaxing, and educative.

As we embrace change with open hearts and psyches, we find that the journey of aging isn't a destination but a continuous evolution toward greater vitality, wisdom, and satisfaction. With resilience, boldness, and adaptability as our guiding stars, we embark on the journey of being forever youthful, writing our account of healthy aging and fulfillment with each step we take.

• Managing stress and Resilience

In the bustling city of Evergreen, where time appeared to stream as quickly as the waterway through its roads, lived an elder named Evelyn. Despite the difficulties life tossed in her direction, Evelyn radiated a sense of calm and resilience that appeared to oppose her age.

Evelyn's mystery lay in her day-to-day routine of mindfulness. Every morning, as the sun cast its brilliant beams upon her garden, she would sit underneath the shade of an old oak tree, her eyes shut in calm thought. With every breath, she let go of the worries, difficulties, and challenges that overburdened her, finding comfort in the gentle rhythm of her heartbeat.

However, Evelyn's journey towards inner peace hadn't always been smooth sailing. In her youthful days, she had been confronted with her share of troubles and challenges - from the loss of friends and family to surprising mishaps in her career. However, with every trial, she discovered a reservoir of strength within herself that she never knew existed.

One particular testing period came when Evelyn chose to resign from her life-long profession as a teacher. For quite a long time, she had emptied her entire being into nurturing young minds, but presently confronted with the possibility of a questionable future, she felt a pang of fear troubling her heart.

However, rather than succumbing to despair, Evelyn decided to embrace the change with grace and resilience. She embarked on a journey of self-discovery, exploring new hobbies, volunteering in her community, and connecting with friends and family. Through it all, she found that genuine satisfaction and happiness didn't come from external trapping of success, but from within- from the relationship she developed, the experiences she appreciated, and the lessons she learnt.

As the years passed, Evelyn's hair turned silver, and her steps grew slower, but her spirit remained forever youthful - vibrant, curious, and full of life. She had discovered that resilience wasn't about staying away from stress or difficulty, but rather facing them head-on with courage and conviction. In doing so, she had opened the way to aging and maturing gracefully - not just in the body, but in mind and spirit too.

• *Coping with Transitions*

Change was a constant companion in the town of Evergreen, where the seasons moved like the pages of a very worn book, every part bringing its delights and distresses. But, as far as some might be concerned, the change starting with one time of life and then onto the next was met with fear and vulnerability.

Such was the situation for Sarah, a new retiree who ended up at a crossroads as she bid goodbye to the recognizable rhythms of her profession and wandered into the unknown domain of retirement. For a long time, Sarah had defined herself by her profession, finding purpose and fulfillment in her job. Presently, confronted with the possibility of an unfilled schedule and vast days extending before her, she felt a feeling of unease settling in her heart.

However, Sarah was not one to shrink from a challenge. Still up in the air to embrace this new phase of her life with open arms, she set out on a journey to find what gave her joy and satisfaction. She delved into her passion, reconnecting with long-lost leisure hobbies and interests she had set aside in the bustle and hustle of her career.

Along the way, Sarah experienced startling open doors and fortunate experiences that reinvigorated her days. From joining a neighborhood planting club to chipping in at a nearby animal shelter, she found a sense of purpose and belonging

that she never realized was missing.

However, amid the excitement of her newfound adventure, Sarah couldn't shake off the lingering sense of loss that accompanied the end of her career. It was as if she was expressing farewell to a close friend - recognizable, soothing, but then touched with a hint of bitterness.

However, as the seasons changed and the scene of Evergreen changed before her eyes, Sarah came to understand that life was not about sticking to the past or being afraid of the future, but about embracing the present moment with great enthusiasm. She figured out how to see changes not as endings, but rather as fresh starts - amazing chances to develop, improve, and embrace the infinite possibilities that lay ahead.

● Flexibility and Adaptability

In the heart of Evergreen, where the streets hummed with the chatters of birds and the chuckling of youngsters, lived a wise elder named Elias. With his weathered hands and sparkling eyes, Elias was a pillar of strength and resilience in his community, a living demonstration of the force of adaptability and flexibility despite change.

Since the beginning, Elias has figured out how to navigate life's twists and turns with grace and ease. Experiencing childhood in a little town settled amid the mountains, he had seen firsthand the consistently changing rhythms of nature - the moving seasons, the back-and-forth movement of the tides, the dance of light and shadow across the landscape.

These examples of versatility and adaptability served Elias well all through his life, from his days as a youthful rancher keeping an eye on the fields to his later years as a darling senior in the town of Evergreen. Whether confronted with a bombed crop, an unexpected tempest, or a difficult choice, Elias moved toward every obstruction with a feeling of strength and cleverness, finding creative solutions where others saw only roadblocks. One particularly memorable instance came when Elias chose to set out on a journey to explore the world past the lines of Evergreen. Furnished with only a solid strolling stick and an insatiable curiosity, he set out on a grand adventure, navigating mountains, crossing waterways, and wandering into the unknown depths of the wilderness

On his way, Elias experienced several difficulties and hindrances - from misleading territory to surprising experiences with wild animals. But, through everything, he stayed unflinching in his assurance to adjust and survive, drawing upon his inner reserves of strength and shrewdness to explore the consistently changing landscape of his journey.

As the sun plunged underneath the skyline and the stars glimmered above, Elias ended up remaining on a desolate slope, looking out at the huge span of the world spread out before him. At that time, he understood that life was not tied in with sticking to the familiar and fearing the unknown but about embracing change with great enthusiasm and a willing heart.

For Elias, the journey was not just a physical one, but also that of the soul - a journey towards self-discovery, growth, and satisfaction. Furthermore, as he remained underneath the shade of stars, encompassed by the magnificence and miracle of the world, he realized that regardless of where lives might lead, he would continuously be directed by the ageless insight of flexibility and adaptability, forever young in spirit and unwavering in strength.

*

As we embrace change with open hearts and brains, we find that the journey of maturing isn't a destination but a continuous evolution toward vitality, wisdom, and satisfaction. With flexibility, mental courage, and adaptability as our guiding stars, we set out on the experience of being forever youthful, writing our own story of health maturing and satisfaction with each step we take.

Chapter Six

Embracing Aging with Elegance and Gratitude.

Dear adventurers of all ages, from the youthful and spirited to the wise and seasoned,

As we venture through the embroidery of life, we are reminded that aging isn't a destination but a natural and inseparable aspect of the human experience. Yet, apart from being a weight to be feared or kept away from, aging is a gift to be embraced with effortlessness and appreciation, a journey of self-discovery, growth, and fulfillment.

In our quest for eternal youthfulness and vitality, we have explored diverse ways by which we can nourish our bodies, psyches, and spirits, weaving together practical wisdom and timeless truth to create a guide for healthy aging and fulfillment. From establishing healthy habits and routines to implementing self-care strategies and setting meaningful goals, we have uncovered the keys to unlocking the fountain of youthfulness that resides inside every one of us regardless of age.

But, beyond the physical and substantial aspect of aging lies a more profound truth - that true youthfulness isn't estimated by the quantity of candles on our birthday cake or the wrinkles on our skin, but by the vitality of our spirit, the resilience of our heart, and the profundity of our gratitude for the endowment of life itself.

All in all, how would we embrace aging with grace and gratitude? It starts with a change in perspective, an acknowledgment that each phase of life brings its exceptional gifts and opens doors for growth. Similarly, as the changing seasons bring new colors to the landscape and new adventures to be had, so too does each passing year offer us the opportunity to grow, learn relearn, and love more deeply than ever before.

For the children among us, aging is a wondrous journey of discovery, an opportunity to explore the world with wide-eyed wonder and insatiable curiosity. As you develop and learn, make sure to cherish every second, for time elapses quickly, and soon you will find yourself embarking on your adventures of self-discovery and growth.

For teenagers and young adults aging is a period of change and self-discovery, an opportunity to spread your wings and soar higher to new heights and possibilities. Embrace the difficulties and experiences that come your way, realizing that each experience is a stepping stone on the path to becoming the person you're meant to be.

For the young at heart, aging is a period of renewal and reinvention, a chance to rediscover interests long neglected and seek after dreams yet unrealized. Embrace the wisdom of your years and the richness of your experiences, realizing that age isn't a hindrance however an honorable badge, a testament to a life well lived and a spirit well loved.

What's more, for the elders among us, aging is a period of reflection and gratitude, a chance to enjoy the memories of a lifetime and share the wisdom of the ages with the generation and individuals who come later. Embrace every day as a valuable gift, realizing that your heritage lives on in the hearts and brains of those you have touched along the way.

In the end, embracing aging with grace and gratitude isn't about defying the passage of time but enjoying every moment with joy, eating right, and doing the needful. It is about finding joy in the pleasure of each day, showing gratitude for the blessings that surround us, and peace in the knowledge that we are exactly where we are intended to be, at this time, at this moment.

So let us raise a toast to the adventure of aging, to the journey of self-discovery and growth, and to the beauty of embracing life with open arms and a thankful heart. For in the end, it is not the years in our lives that count but the life in our years, and the legacy of love and laughter that we leave behind for generations to come.

A well-nourished, incorporated with exercises, healthy dieting, physical involvement, and agility is a youthful and vibrant life.

Here's to healthy aging with youthfulness, not just that of the body but also your spirit and soul.